Obesity and Hormones:

Corrective Diets for women

By

Barbara L. Miller

TABLE OF CONTENT

INTRODUCTION

While hormones are important constituents of all living things, the female human species has a very deep connection to these chemical messengers that cause life-changing experiences. Throughout their existence, women go through a myriad of transformations that include but are not limited to puberty, pregnancy, and menopause. From menstruation to menopause, hormonal cycles can have a profound effect on their lives. Hormonal imbalances are becoming increasingly common, with studies indicating that as many as 80% of women experience symptoms of hormonal imbalance at some point in their lives.

The effects of hormonal imbalances can be far-reaching and can manifest in a variety of ways. For instance, some researchers have linked hormonal imbalances to weight gain, depression, anxiety, mood swings, fatigue, and sleep disturbances. One novel discovery found a connection between hormonal imbalance and increased risk of chronic diseases such as type 2 diabetes, cardiovascular disease, and certain cancers.

Unregulated hormones can also affect mental health. The Psychiatrist, Margaret Altemus recently established a relationship between hormonal imbalances in the developmental and adult stages of life to the onset of psychiatric issues later in life.

The good news is that hormonal imbalances can often be corrected through dietary and lifestyle changes. Resetting your hormones through a targeted diet can help to alleviate symptoms and improve overall health. Scientist, Peter F. Foley asserted that a low-carbohydrate diet can improve insulin sensitivity and reduce the risk of type 2 diabetes.

Another study by a seasoned researcher linked a Mediterranean-style diet, rich in healthy fats and vegetables, to reduced inflammation and mood improvement. In this book, we will delve into the fascinating world of women's hormones and explore how they impact our bodies and minds.

We will examine the latest research on hormonal imbalances and its associated health risks, as well as provide practical strategies for resetting your hormones through diet and lifestyle changes. This author desires to empower women with the knowledge and tools they need to take control of their hormonal health and achieve optimal well-being.

CHAPTER 1
The physical Impact of hormones and food, on women's health

The human body is an intricate machine that never fails to inspire awe with its design and engineering. Much like a well-designed car, it requires intelligent signaling mechanisms to operate efficiently.

To help you fully appreciate the smart nature of the human body, think about the warning signals installed on your car dashboard. The eye-catching colors of these signals alert the driver to potential dangers by hinting at different risk levels. While green lights indicate no cause for concern, yellow signals suggest a potential threat that requires immediate action to avert danger. Finally, red signals portend inevitable hazards.

Our bodies have similar mechanisms that keep us informed about our health status, enabling us to take appropriate action when necessary.

We should be grateful for these life-saving prompts and their intelligent modes of operation.

While studying to become a Biochemist, I was always fascinated by the way hormones functioned. My love for automobiles led me to draw a correlation between hormones and car warning signals. But if you are business inclined, you might think of hormones as managers that are delegated by directors to regulate the activities of employees in different departments.

In scientific terms, hormones are chemical messengers that are integral to the functioning of living things. They are produced in specific areas of the body and dispatched to target organs, where they exert their regulatory influence.

We cannot talk about hormones without mentioning the endocrine glands, which are a collection of cells that make and release hormones in response to specific physiological signals. These endocrine glands produce a range of hormones, including testosterone, dopamine, growth hormone, prolactin, and luteinizing hormone.

The hormones live in and perform their duties in body sites like the brain, thyroid, and reproductive organs. For instance, the brain's hypothalamus synthesizes dopamine and the growth hormone. So, hormones represent the face of regulation in the exciting dance of bodily functions, ensuring that everything is in balance and working as it should.

From teenage age to adulthood, women undergo complex changes that involve hormones. The menstrual cycle, ovulation, and pregnancy are well-known examples of body metabolisms whose success depends on hormonal activities. In addition to these, food cravings, mood swings, and skin diseases such as acne are also strongly associated with hormones.

So, as a woman who is intentional about her health, you need to understand how the different hormones in the body function and how these could affect your general well-being. Being mindful of your food intake will also go a long way in ensuring that certain hormones are not triggered to over- or under-production with harmful consequences on both ends.

Over the years, many 'experts' have recommended several measures to manage optimal health in women through food. Some of them advise women to fast, drink slimming teas or eliminate carbohydrates and fat from their diets. The majority of persons who implemented these extreme directions ended up with worse results that further upset their hormonal balance. But apart from these self-imposed experts, there was a time – a decade or two ago, when the scientific understanding of weight loss measures was not right.

It was believed then, that fatty foods must be avoided while maintaining the same carbohydrate intake levels. However, new insights have led to better clarifications. If weight loss is your goal, you need to consider evidence-based results that are proven to work. These principles have been tested and shown to produce positive changes. In the course of this book, the right forms of diet are recommended for women who wish to enjoy some stability and prolong their lives.

Abnormal hormones and your self-confidence

In addition to the internal health dangers that unbalanced hormones can pose to health, there is also the aspect of physical appearance that affects the self-esteem of women.

For instance, acne can become a recurring battle if the root cause, sometimes linked to hormones, is not addressed. Obesity is another tormentor that not only functions as a precursor to many heart diseases but can also alter the physical form of women and their perception by others.

A 2018 study by the National Health and Nutrition Examination Survey (NHANES) pegged the percentage of obese American women at 27.5% out of a total of 61.6% overweight adults. Unhealthy eating habits constitute a notable source of this outcome. In 2020, "Trust for America's Health" produced data that shows an improvement in obesity count as 41.9% of the nation's adults were now reported to be obese. However, this figure represented a 31% increase in adult obesity since 1999.

To better understand the topic of obesity, you need to know how food is digested and absorbed by the organs of the body. A refined understanding of body metabolism will help you see the folly behind some popular anti-obesity advice. This will also prevent you from denying the body the essential nutrients that are necessary for sustaining life.

The female body is delicate, so any lifestyle change that must be effected should be done with utmost care. Moving with the trend is not ideal because, even though we have the same organs, our genetic makeup accounts for our uniqueness. There is a clear and strong bond between food, hormones, and female health.

Instead of providing a personalized plan, this book aims to help you understand the process of sugar and fat metabolism and the ideal principles that should guide your adoption of healthy meal plans. It will also help you see which hormone is responsible for a given manifestation and how to keep it under control.

Aside from these, the toxins in the environment are relatively obscure actors that also contaminate the diet and health of women. Pesticides, laced in foods purchased from grocery stores, contain inordinate amounts of chemicals that might upset the normal hormonal balance and damage vital organs of the body.

In most environments, issues such as gas flaring, climate change, and pollution also contribute to the number of unhealthy substances that women are exposed to. How about the numerous personal care products on the shelves of many homes? When used indiscriminately, these could upset the pH of the skin and extract unusual responses from the body.

Appropriate diet that can help you thrive during your menstrual cycle

The menstrual cycle is a complex and often challenging experience for many women. The first phase, known as the follicular phase, is marked by the arrival of our monthly flow.

This stage involves shedding the uterine lining and can last for approximately three to six days, leaving many women feeling tired, sluggish, and experiencing painful cramps. What is to be blamed for these emotional and physical changes? Fluctuating hormones, of course. At this stage, progesterone and estrogen levels are at their lowest, which explains the low energy and overall sluggishness that many women tend to feel. So, what can be done from a nutritional standpoint to ease the effects of this phase?

First and foremost, it is crucial to increase your intake of iron-rich foods. Iron is a vital mineral that helps produce red blood cells and transports oxygen throughout the body. Due to menstrual blood losses, iron deficiency is one of the most common nutritional deficiencies among women of childbearing age.

Low iron levels during menstruation also explain why women typically have low energy and fatigue. Therefore, women must compensate for the amount of blood being lost from their period by eating more iron-rich foods during this time.

Animal sources of iron include red meat, poultry, and fish, while plant-based sources include fortified cereals, tofu, beans, lentils, and other legumes.

Another essential nutrient to consider during this phase is vitamin C. Not only is it an antioxidant that helps with immunity, healthy skin, and wound healing, it also helps our bodies absorb iron even better. Think of vitamin C as a helper that boosts the effectiveness of iron. Therefore, if you are adding an iron-rich meal during that time of the month, make sure to pair it with a source of vitamin C, such as citrus fruits or vegetables like bell peppers, tomatoes, or leafy greens.

On the other hand, inhibitors present in coffee and caffeinated teas, green and black tea can interfere with iron absorption. These beverages contain polyphenols, an antioxidant substance that decreases the amount of iron the body absorbs. Moreover, caffeine is a vasoconstrictor, meaning it makes the blood vessels in your body constrict. This constriction can make period cramps even worse for many women.

Therefore, it is best to stick to normal tea on those first few days or, at the very least, spread the caffeine out at least an hour before or after your iron-rich meal to help maximize the absorption of iron.

As for food, it is wise to stay nourished with lighter, less processed meals. Salt increases water retention, which causes bloating, and fatty foods increase prostaglandin production, which can increase contractions or cramps.

Focusing on recipes with lots of veggies and fruits, especially those that are rich in hydrating water and energizing carbs, may help with your fading energy levels. Also, incorporating whole grains and legumes will be beneficial. Meals during this phase do not need to compulsorily please your taste buds but should be healthy foods that are rich in nutrients. Simplicity is key, focusing on whole ingredients whenever possible.

Finally, a little light, gentle exercise may play a therapeutic role in relieving cramps by releasing endorphins, which help improve mood and relax the body. Exercise may also provide a distraction from the discomfort of the cramps, which is always a good thing. The exercise does not have to be tedious but light and suited to your circumstance.

The ovulation phase marks the beginning of a new egg's preparation for its descent down the fallopian tubes to the uterus. During this phase, there is an increase in estrogen, testosterone, follicle-stimulating hormone, and luteinizing hormone, which explains the increase in energy levels and libido that we feel. This is an excellent time to move and exercise as energy levels are balanced.

You could hit the gym for some weight training, or even a spin class. As women, we are also built to be in the best frame for having sex during this phase. The higher energy levels and brighter moods are a perfect match for moderate to high-intensity activities.

It is also a good time to work in the kitchen and prepare meals as this phase allows for optimal energy levels. You can explore the kitchen by cooking protein-rich meals, soups, and vegetables for yourself and your family.

The third phase is the luteal phase which happens when ovulation does not result in fertilization, and hormone levels decline. During this phase, women experience premenstrual syndrome, which may include symptoms such as cramps, headaches, bloating, mood swings, fatigue, and food cravings.

Women also have increased cravings for sweet, carb-rich foods during the luteal phase, as research has shown that food cravings are linked to the amount of leptin in our blood, and leptin is the hunger hormone that tells us when we are full.

It is important to listen to our bodies and notice any patterns that arise during this phase to assess what our bodies need. We should also allow ourselves to have carbohydrates during this phase, as research suggests that we tend to crave refined carbs. However, we should focus on slow-burning, delicious carbs and pair them with a source of protein and fat to keep blood sugar levels balanced.

We should also increase our fiber intake during this phase to ease constipation, as progesterone levels are at an all-time high right before our period. This can be achieved by consuming fiber-rich whole grains, berries, vegetables, flax, beans, and nuts. Finally, it is important to focus on fresh foods instead of highly processed, salty foods during this phase, as these can cause more gas and discomfort.

Key nutrients for hormonal health

Balancing hormones can be challenging, but certain foods can make a difference. Nuts and seeds like almonds, pumpkin seeds, and sunflower seeds are rich in magnesium, which can help reduce premenstrual syndrome symptoms and improve mood. Cruciferous vegetables like broccoli, kale, and cauliflower are packed with compounds that support liver detoxification, and this helps to balance estrogen levels.

Also, omega-3-rich foods such as salmon, chia seeds, and flax seeds can reduce inflammation and regulate menstrual cycles. Raspberries are abundant in antioxidants that can reduce inflammation and support hormonal balance.

Another great source of healthy fats that is crucial for hormone production and balance is avocado. Beta-sitosterol is found in this delicious fruit and this substance has been studied for its ability to reduce stress by acting on the hormone, cortisol. Incorporating these foods into your diet can be a natural and effective way to balance your hormones.

The role of modern medicine in resolving hormonal problems

The hospitals are often flooded with issues related to infertility, polycystic ovary syndrome (PCOS), and endometriosis. While it is true that these problems could have genetic causes, they might also be the result of certain lifestyle issues like obesity and skewed hormones. High levels of androgen (a male sex hormone) in women have also been linked to PCOS. To establish the presence of a hormonal issue, women ought to consult a doctor for proper diagnosis.

The hormonal profile test is often requested by medical doctors when they want to establish an abnormality in a woman's hormones. These tests give a true picture of the situation and will eventually help determine the exact factor the woman should be targeting.

To achieve success when dealing with hormone issues, knowledge of what is right and balanced should be the prime goal. You should strive to consume a balanced diet instead of eliminating nutritive foods. Also, monitoring blood sugar levels will prevent a sudden, uncontrollable change that will be difficult to manage.

Dietary approaches like the Mediterranean and ketogenic diets have been tested and certified by authorities in nutrition to normalize body metabolism. We will delve into these feeding styles to understand the principles behind them and just how they will aid you in achieving your diet and health goals. First, let us examine how hormones cause weight-related issues.

CHAPTER 2
Unraveling the relationship between Hormones and Women's Body Size

To get a true picture of how hormones affect the weight of women, we need to first pinpoint the exact hormones that are associated with weight, how they work, and measures for managing them.

Estrogen is a class of female sex hormones that determine the state of a woman's reproductive and sexual health. This name serves as a general umbrella for hormones such as estradiol, estriol, and estrone. Estrogen is produced in the ovaries, the adrenal gland, and the adipose (fat) cells. It can also be found in male blood and semen. In women, it regulates the menstrual cycle, the production of the secondary female sex features, pregnancy, mood, bone formation, eating habits, and lactation.

Since we have set our sights on body size, we will dwell more on estrogen's contribution to weight. The hypothalamus is a coordinating brain part where the estrogen hormone is produced. This hormone acts on some nerve cells to limit the amount of food you eat and increase physical activity and the distribution of fat. The type of fat distribution that is engineered by moderate estrogen levels is the positive type.

Women acquire a pear shape that results from allocating more fat to the hip areas than to the abdomen and upper body. Therefore, if estrogen levels reduce, there will be more food intake and the accumulation of fat, a large portion of which is unhealthy. For menopausal women, the fat accumulation is noticeable around the abdomen.

Now you may wonder what factors might cause a decline in estrogen levels. Naturally, estrogen has been proven to decrease when women approach menopause. So, there is a greater chance of accumulating abdominal fat deposits at this stage in life.

In addition to menopause, some cancer medications (the aromatase inhibitors) and therapies, excessive amounts of exercise, and oophorectomy (the removal of one or two ovaries) are culprits of estrogen decrease. Eating disorders such as bulimia nervosa cause food binging and a resultant drop in estrogen levels. If you have or are undergoing any of these conditions, you should keep an eye on your estrogen levels.

Progesterone and weight management

Progesterone is a steroid hormone that is produced by the corpus luteum of a woman's ovary, and it is responsible for regulating menstruation and pregnancy. The hormone is produced with the prospect of implantation and pregnancy because it strengthens the lining of the ovaries; if the expected implantation fails to occur, the lining is shed and menstruation occurs. Suppose a woman gets pregnant; more progesterone is produced to enable pregnancy.

The relationship between progesterone and body size is not a direct one; however, there is still a need for close monitoring.

After ovulation, the level of progesterone produced by the body begins to build up. Then, there is a corresponding rise in the amount of energy used for metabolism. Chances are that the body will need more food from which it can tap some energy to support body metabolism.

Excessive consumption of food during this period may cause an increase in body weight. So, instead of throwing caution to the wind, your diet should be at its best to avoid any unwanted changes in weight and appearance.

Hormonal changes during pregnancy and the impact on body composition

During pregnancy, women undergo significant physiological changes, particularly in the levels and functions of hormones such as estrogen and progesterone.

These hormonal shifts do more than just influence mood; they also have an important influence on pregnancy and physical activity. Estrogen and progesterone are the primary hormones of pregnancy, with levels that increase significantly throughout gestation.

Progesterone levels become extraordinarily high during pregnancy, leading to the relaxation of ligaments and joints throughout the body. This hormone is also responsible for stretching the uterus so that it can carry a fetus. Progesterone causes internal structures, such as the ureters that connect the kidneys to the bladder, to increase in size.

The surge in estrogen levels during pregnancy helps to improve vascularization and support the developing fetus by supplying more essential vitamins to them. Additionally, estrogen is believed to play a critical role in fetal development and maturation.

As estrogen levels steadily increase throughout pregnancy, they reach their peak in the third trimester. The increase in estrogen levels during pregnancy triggers nausea and during the second trimester, estrogen is heavily involved in the development of milk ducts that enlarge the breasts.

Due to the physical changes that women experience during pregnancy, they may become greatly limited in their ability to exercise and this eventually results in weight gain. The negative effect of such weight gain is that it increases the workload on the body and slows down the circulation of blood and bodily fluids, leading to swelling in the limbs and face.

This fluid retention contributes significantly to the weight gain experienced during pregnancy. To successfully manage swelling during pregnancy, it is vital to take enough rest, avoid long periods of standing, reduce the consumption of caffeine and sodium intake, and increase dietary potassium. Overall, understanding the hormonal and physical changes that occur during pregnancy can help women navigate this unique and transformative experience with greater ease and confidence.

Important weight markers to consider

It may be hard to link hormones to certain diseases if there is no clinical result yet. But if a woman is already diagnosed with certain health conditions like PCOS and insulin resistance, it will be more accurate to attribute her sudden weight gain to these problems.

Polycystic Ovarian Syndrome (PCOS) is diagnosed when there is an excessive amount of male androgens. This prevents the hormones responsible for producing the follicle-stimulating hormone from performing their jobs properly.

When this happens, the woman cannot produce eggs for fertilization. It is, therefore, not surprising that this condition is responsible for infertility in women. Increased production of body hair and acne are additional signs of PCOS, and the type of weight gain that manifests in PCOS patients is the abdominal type.

This kind of fat is not easy to lose and could be a precursor to many deadly respiratory issues. Some signs that may be telling of thecondition include irregular menstruation and the presence of polycystic ovaries seen during an imaging test.

Let us now examine insulin and its role in weight gain. Insulin is a hormone that regulates the usage of glucose and the conversion of glucose to energy. When insulin is unable to execute its normal regulatory functions, an excessive amount of blood sugar results followed by a rise in androgen levels.

Today, certain lifestyles can predispose one to insulin resistance. A sedentary lifestyle restricts slow fat burning in the liver and abdomen. Also, the overwhelming acceptance of processed meals can dismantle the normal glucose levels of individuals who resort to unsupervised food consumption. Once again, the importance of balance in food choices is brought to the fore.

Thyroid and cortisol are next to be evaluated for their regulatory functions. When some disruptions in the normal flow of the body's systems affect these hormones, weight gain is often a commonly associated effect. The thyroid hormone maintains the rate of metabolism in the body.

Low thyroid levels result in a condition known as hypothyroidism, while a high thyroid level is called hyperthyroidism. If the thyroid level is low, this means that the body's ability to extract energy from the food substances it consumes has diminished. More water and salt can be retained as a result of this development. This is why hypothyroid patients tend to add some weight.

Next, stress from daily activities can also cause added weight. After a busy day at work, the body becomes exhausted and it may be wise to take some rest. However, some people have become so invested in the pursuit of their goals that they hardly take some time off for quality rest.

The gloomy fate that awaits a machine continually used with little or no maintenance will soon apply to the human body that makes no provision for rest. An upswing in cortisol levels is linked to stress, and when unmanaged, there could be a ripple of ugly outcomes.

You may want to know what causes the production of cortisol. The hypothalamus has been previously described as a part of the brain responsible for controlling certain important functions in the body. When the body is in a state of unrest, some signals are sent to the hypothalamus, which produces cortisol and adrenaline. Cortisol increases blood sugar levels, which allows the person under some form of stress to stay alert while coping with the situation.

However, while cortisol stimulates the production of sugar, it slows the metabolism of the digestive system. Now, you can guess how weight gain results. The inability of the body to metabolize food and transform it into energy as a result of cortisol's regulatory function translates to weight gain.

So, here we have it. Hormones are designed to switch on and off based on the body's present state. Even though we have these important regulators for sustaining life, we need to avoid extreme conditions that can trigger weight gain. In addition to monitoring weight and the causes of obesity, knowledge of hormones will also help pinpoint why other health challenges like polycystic ovarian syndrome, infertility, acne, and irregular menstrual cycles occur.

Many have suggested different diets as measures to shed weight but ketogenic diets stand out for their hormone-stabilizing effects. In the next chapter, we will consider what this diet consists of and how it can be effectively used to normalize hormone function.

CHAPTER 3
The Enigma of Ketogenic Diets

Often, individuals on a quest to find a hormone-friendly diet do not know so much about the ketogenic diet. I was also puzzled the first time I heard about this diet and the kinds of foods that ensure compliance.

A lady who was on a mission to shed post-delivery weight once described the ketogenic diet as using fat to kill fat, and this pretty much explains the nature of this diet.

A ketogenic diet requires you to eat a minimal amount of carbohydrates and a large portion of high-fat foods. The aim is to condition the body into utilizing its fat instead of sugar for energy metabolism.

After some time, the body begins to experience ketosis because of the reduced sugar levels, which are accompanied by a reduction in insulin levels. Instead of glucose, the brain also starts to use ketones as its source of energy.

This diet has been proven to generate a considerable reduction in weight for most people. An investigation by Gordana Markovikj indicated a 50-pound mean weight loss for women who participated in the study. Over an average of 78.2 days, the male participants lost 65.5 pounds.

The effectiveness of this diet has been demonstrated in many other studies. Another study that combined the benefits of a ketogenic diet and the introduction of a Mediterranean diet also produced a result that indicated an average 10 percent loss in weight with no relapse after 12 months.

The additional beauty of this diet lies in its ability to target the hormones that stimulate hunger. Ghrelin and insulin are some of these hunger-inducing hormones whose activities are stalled by the mechanisms of a ketogenic diet.

Also, satiety is a side benefit of a high-fat diet plan. Because fatty foods are slower to digest, they make you feel fuller and less likely to consume excessive food portions. These benefits are necessary for weight control.

Getting it right on a ketogenic diet requires maintaining the body's supply of other nutrients. Proteins are important constituents of a ketogenic diet but many fruits will need to be cut off. This might be surprising, but the reason is not far-fetched because most fruits contain a high amount of carbohydrates. The standard ketogenic diet consists of 70% fat, 20% protein, and 10% carbohydrate; however, there could be mild alterations to these specifications.

How the ketogenic diet corrects hormonal issues

Most of the hormonal issues ravaging women today can be managed with a ketogenic meal plan. Estrogen, progesterone, and many other hormones are produced through the metabolism of fat. Since a keto-based meal plan promotes the consumption of healthy fat, the body will be prompted to produce these hormones in optimal amounts that support health.

When estrogen spirals out of control before menstruation, women experience acne, cramps, agitation, fatigue, and other unwholesome effects. Excessive consumption of sugar stimulates fat cells that turn over more estrogen. A keto meal plan keeps estrogen in check by regulating sugar levels.

The inclusion of green vegetables and herbs will also clear toxic elements that could result in the overproduction of some hormones. Individuals managing polycystic ovarian syndrome also tap into these positive results. If they follow this diet, they would improve fertility and induce weight loss.

Cortisol's presence in the body can also be regulated with the right diet regimen. When the human body is stressed, cortisol stimulates more sugar production and reduces concentration on normal body functions like reproduction. So, a rise in sugar levels is accompanied by a dip in estrogen, progesterone, and other sex hormones, but a good keto diet can prevent this.

Getting started on a ketogenic diet

For almost every significant change we make in life, the body usually needs some time for full adaptation. Similarly, when you are new to the ketogenic diet, it might also take some time before your body accepts this new form of feeding. Three important steps that can help you when you are just starting include eating keto-compliant meals, eating these meals in the right proportions, and managing the infamous keto flu.

To kick start and sustain ketosis, carbohydrate-dense foods ought to be replaced with protein- and fat-rich meals. Your go-to options, in this case, will include leafy vegetables, dairy products, keto-friendly sweeteners, seeds, nuts, high-fat meats, and healthy oils.

Foods that must be avoided in their entirety include grains, starchy meals, high-carb fruits, and sugar. You also need to develop the skill of reading food labels to understand the nutritional content of these foods and ways to substitute unapproved meals for the compliant kinds.

Knowing how much of the right foods to eat is another vital step in beginning a successful keto journey. With a digital device or the good old paper and pen, you can track the percentage of carbohydrates, proteins, and fats that you are consuming each day. Some online resources have automated calculators that can help you check your daily consumption.

The keto lifestyle should dominate every aspect of your life so that while you write your budget, plan your meal, or develop food recipes, only keto-friendly items will be given precedence. Remember, the goal is to have just 10% of your total daily calories come from carbohydrates.

Lastly, the keto flu is a common side effect of the ketogenic diet. Common symptoms include fatigue, burnout, and slowed brain activity. To keep these effects in check, make it a priority to drink lots of water, get enough sleep, and keep electrolytes like sodium and potassium in check.

Also, you need to regularly monitor markers like blood pressure, blood glucose, and lipid levels to be sure that there are no odd results. If you feel sick at any time, consult your doctor for medical help.

The objective is to get started and maintain the lifestyle, hence the need to follow proven steps for sustainability. There are more chances of sticking to this diet plan if tenable measures like those above are adhered to.

Meal Planning and Preparation Tips

Some individuals have special considerations when it comes to diet. While the dairy-focused plan is acceptable to some people, others prefer a vegetable-based plan. The healthy and dirty keto diets are also two key routes that some take to achieve their weight loss goals.

The debate over keto diets rages on, with many proponents championing the benefits of a healthy keto diet over a dirty one. The former prioritizes nutrient-rich foods, including leafy greens, vegetables, and healthy fats, while limiting carbs, but the latter simply focus on keeping carbohydrates at bay.

By following the healthy approach, individuals can get more benefits like improved insulin resistance, more feelings of satisfaction, and a better physical appearance.

A healthy keto diet consists of 5 to 10% carbs (including veggies), 20% protein, and 70% fat, whereas dirty keto allows for more carbohydrate consumption. The emphasis on vegetables in healthy keto is because of the vitamins, minerals, and phytonutrients they offer.

As you start a keto meal, it is recommended to begin by skipping breakfast, combining two meals within a six-hour window, and adding more fat to reduce the need for snacking. After you become more adapted, you can reduce fat and focus on foods such as pasture-raised eggs, shellfish, sardines, organic meats, and olives.

Nuts and seeds are good options for some people, but those prone to kidney stones should be careful with almonds and spinach. While cheese can be incorporated, it should be consumed in moderation, preferably grass-fed and organic. In summary, beginners can get off on a good footing with a basic and nutrient-dense ketogenic plan.

Tracking Progress and Hormonal Changes

Contrary to misconceptions about the negative impact of the ketogenic diet and intermittent fasting on women's hormones, objective scientific views show that hormonal health in women is greatly improved on a keto plan.

When you commence a ketogenic diet, you can gauge your progress by evaluating the state of your hormones. You will record many benefits if you religiously adhere to a healthy keto diet. First, the reduction of insulin levels will enhance fat-burning hormones like the growth hormone, thyroid, adrenaline, and glucagon. The presence of these hormones, will, in turn, quicken the weight loss process.

A diet rich in fat stimulates the production of steroid hormones like estrogen, progesterone, cortisol, and testosterone.

In addition to hormone production, this meal plan guarantees hormone balance as a side benefit. Furthermore, consuming healthy fats will also increase bile production by activating the thyroid hormone and allowing the absorption of fat-soluble vitamins like vitamins A, D, and E.

The balance achieved through a good keto diet helps women with PCOS reach normal androgen levels. It also facilitates brain repair and growth and improves fertility and libido.

Despite all of these positive possibilities, it is also possible to record negative results after some time of following a keto meal plan. However, the result that you get depends on the type of keto plan that you are practicing. With a dirty keto diet, one may experience irregular menstrual cycles, a decrease in libido, or abnormal hormone levels.

Ugly outcomes can also arise from fasting too much or just not striving for balance in the adoption of this regimen.

Side effects and the importance of seeking professional advice

When choosing a diet, it is crucial to consider its long-term effects on health rather than focusing solely on short-term benefits. While restricted diets like ketogenic or low-carbohydrate diets may help with weight loss, they pose a risk of vitamin deficiency and fiber and phytonutrient deprivation.

To manage these potential side effects, vegetables should be a regular feature in your meals. Remember that while you can get these vitamins from supplements, food remains the most ideal source of essential vitamins.

Additionally, high-fat diets can lead to glucose intolerance and insulin resistance, causing health issues like fatty liver and kidney stones. This side effect can be managed by avoiding excessive sodium consumption. Ideally, you should not consume more than 2500 mg per day. People who are at risk of developing kidney stones must drink up to 3 liters of water daily.

More so, clinical studies have shown that the ketogenic diet results in fat-free mass loss and thus increases the likelihood of dehydration. This further stresses the need for water consumption.

Another negative outcome of high-fat diets is linked to increased LDL cholesterol, which is harmful to heart health. This can be curtailed by eating only when hungry, avoiding processed foods, and opting for more unsaturated fat foods like avocados, vegetables, and fish.

Studies show that these keto-compliant meals have LDL-lowering effects. Therefore, it is essential to choose a keto diet that considers overall health benefits and involves nutrient-dense foods.

The ketogenic diet is excellent for many health goals. To fight obesity and counteract certain hormonal disruptions, this diet can prove to be a good remedy. However, if you have any serious medical conditions, it is wise to contact a medical professional for the best way to adopt a weight-reduction plan.

CHAPTER 4
Detoxification and the Mediterranean diet

In our environments, we are constantly exposed to toxic substances that are inimical to our health. The cars on the streets release harmful carbon monoxide, which is a leading cause of pollution, and so is the case with our home air conditioners that emit harmful chlorofluorocarbons.

These not only have the capacity to damage our immediate environment but also the ozone layer. Certain lifestyle choices and health conditions encourage the buildup of toxins. When you realize the need to switch to a better dietary plan, such as the ketogenic diet or the Mediterranean diet, it is also important that you support the body's detoxification process.

Supporting the detoxification process prepares the body for the digestive activities that are launched during a metabolic condition like ketogenesis. For example, when fat is broken down during ketogenesis, toxins can be released into the blood-stream, but this becomes more pronounced when the body is just transitioning from a carbohydrate-focused plan to a fat-degrading one. To prevent conflicting results, you should learn to detoxify your body by following accurate detoxification procedures.

Detoxification involves ridding the body of toxins and harmful substances that endanger health. As earlier explained, many things in our environments predispose us to the risk of accumulating waste materials. If you are observant, signals such as fatigue, headache, constipation, and obesity might also be telling signs of the need to detoxify.

After detoxification, the body tends to operate at its best. There will also be an improved rate of brain repair, boosted energy levels, a better immune system, smoother skin, and bodily functions that proceed in a faster and more optimal manner.

A primary organ responsible for detoxification in the body is the liver. After eating, the digestive process commences, and one of the crucial steps is the passage of food materials, and toxins, through the liver. The liver detoxifies harmful substances and sends them to the urine to be disposed of, while the improved materials are returned to the blood.

When toxins are present in large amounts, a lot of pressure is put on the liver to detoxify them, and an eventual case of liver failure may arise. To keep this vital organ in the best condition, there is every need to eat foods that will bolster its condition. Antioxidant-rich meals protect the cells from toxic radicals. You will improve your overall health when you opt for a diet that introduces more of these substances into the digestive tract.

Requirements of a plant-based diet

The Mediterranean diet is a plant-based diet that enriches the body with antioxidants. Its concentration of nuts, vegetables, minimal amounts of dairy, and natural cereals are just what the core body organs need to normalize all abnormalities. This diet is rooted in Greek culture, and olive oil is the main source of oil.

The oil is sourced from the olive tree, and the main benefit it provides stems from its composition of monounsaturated fat. As mentioned before, monounsaturated fat lowers bad cholesterol levels significantly. So, people who use this oil will mostly have reduced exposure to heart diseases, diabetes, stroke, cancer, and obesity.

Another benefit of the Mediterranean diet is its liver-protecting feature. The constituent foods have a fiber-rich content, as seen in dried fruits, grains, and nuts that avail the body with close to 15 grams of vegetable fiber daily.

Vegetables, fruits, red wine, and olive oil, all of which contain minerals, vitamins, carotenoids, and flavonoids prevent oxidative stress. These elements and compounds are touted for their effectiveness in renewing cells damaged by free radicals.

Apart from olive oil, nuts, and seeds, other sources of healthy fat are available in the Mediterranean diet. Fishes like tuna, mackerel, and sardines are rich in polyunsaturated fat, another healthy source of healthy fat.

Those who adopt this diet have more options to feed from and will also record the same or better results compared to other restrictive plans. So, flexibility is one of the perks of a Mediterranean diet.

In addition to general well-being, hormone health thrives under a Mediterranean feeding pattern. Vitamin E present in fish like salmon is necessary for the production of cholesterol, and cholesterol is a precursor to the production of any steroid hormone you can think of. As a reminder, cortisol, progesterone, estradiol, and testosterone are examples of steroid hormones.

Obesity is also well managed with this vitamin because it enhances leptin, a primary hunger controller that also promotes the feeling of fullness.

Selenium, vitamin B, and zinc obtained from shellfish and nuts also help hormone synthesis. Flaxseeds are especially known for stimulating a better form of estrogen called phytoestrogen, which has the potential of reducing conventional estrogen levels in menopausal women.

Developing healthy eating habits

Developing healthy eating patterns is essential for long-term health and wellness. However, it is difficult for some people to establish daily, healthy eating habits. Others might even find themselves constantly switching from one trend to another because they have a vague idea of what they should eat to stay healthy but struggle to follow through with consistency.

So, it is not unusual to feel stressed when making food choices or striving to maintain a healthy balance. There are three essential steps that you can apply to establish personalized healthy eating habits.

First and foremost, you should know what foods to eat to nourish your body. Eating an abundance of plant-based foods (as is obtainable in a Mediterranean diet), rich in essential vitamins, minerals, antioxidants, and nutrients, supports your overall well-being. These foods help keep you full and energized and stabilize your hormones and digestion, among other things.

Studies have also shown that they can improve heart health, reduce inflammation, stabilize blood sugar, and support the immune system. In addition to these, other healthy options like the ketogenic regimen have been researched and marked as excellent for attaining health goals. Whatever choice you make will largely depend on your ideologies and individual health requirements.

Another practical principle that can help you establish consistency is knowing how to eat. Conscious eating is all about eating healthy meals while striving for balance and making room to explore other meals that you love. By becoming more aware of your body signals, hunger cues, satiety cues, and food behaviors, you can make better choices that align with your needs and wants.

Consistency enables you to create healthier eating habits for life by making small changes that improve your relationship with food. It also lets you enjoy nutrient-packed, plant-based, or high-fat, low-carb foods without feeling deprived.

The last principle is focused on creating a sustainable lifestyle of healthy eating habits. This involves planning your meals, mastering basic cooking etiquettes and methods, making smart choices when eating out, and stocking your pantry with wholesome ingredients that allow you to whip up quick and easy meals.

It is also essential to prioritize self-care by making time for activities that reduce stress and promote overall well-being. Given that you have more control over your meals when you prepare them yourself, it is recommended that you learn how to cook and enjoy the process.

By following these three guidelines, you can establish healthy eating habits that are enjoyable, sustainable, and aligned with your personality.

Essential hacks to help you thrive on a Mediterranean diet

If you settle on a Mediterranean diet, you need to get used to the idea of incorporating more fruits and vegetables into your diet. You also have to include healthy fats while eliminating processed foods.

If you dislike vegetables like spinach, kale, onions, and broccoli, you could still get your daily fix of essential nutrients from vegetables by blending them into sweet fruits like bananas, cherries, pears, watermelon, mangoes, and apples. This hack spares you the rigor of chewing vegetables you do not like while directly ingesting all the nutrients that they provide. Also, if you do not like eating some fruits in their natural forms, you could make juices from them.

Modeling the appearance of regular foods after their healthy alternatives is another way to make vegetables more appealing to the eater. For instance, when you crave for cakes, you could mimic the appearance of regular cakes with vegetables. Broccoli, carrots, onions, zucchini, and salt are common ingredients in vegetable cake recipes. It is also possible to get "pasta" from zucchini by grating it in the same spiral form.

In addition, if you wish to fill up your daily dietary consumption with healthy options you could substitute cookies and other snacks with vegetables and nuts. Juices and soups are also ways to consume more vegetables by proxy.

Often, you might have to explore vegetables that you have never tried before to keep the food journey interesting. In most cases, having a regular supply of vegetables will mean that you need to stock up in advance and take advantage of seasons when certain vegetables are in greater supply.

One sign that shows your readiness to follow a healthy eating routine is your willingness to remove processed foods from your diet. This may not be easy as we are surrounded by a vast line-up of refined foods that also seem cheaper when compared to natural foods.

Sure, you love yourself well enough to substitute the temporary ecstasy of sugary foods with the benefits of wholesome living and a prolonged lifespan. Rejecting foods with high sugar content is a good way to limit added sugars found in fizzy drinks, cookies, and other snacks.

Examine ingredient labels to determine the quantity of added sugars and strive to only go for options with minimal sugar content. Instead of sugar, add flavor to food with extracts and spices.

So far, we have seen that detoxification is a very important part of the health journey. The Mediterranean diet is packed full of natural and heart-friendly meals that can help to balance hormones and improve all other aspects of life.

The vitamins, minerals, and antioxidants contained in fruits and vegetables encourage the process of detoxification. We have also seen that detoxification makes it easier for the body to assimilate the workings of a new food regimen.

This way, health goals can be achieved faster. With determination on your part, it will be possible to make these changes. Think of the long-term and immediate benefits that can be gained from these food choices, and stay motivated on the quest to balance your hormones and shed weight without breaking a sweat.

CHAPTER 5
Making a Smooth Switch to Healthy Etiquette

Transitioning from the familiar to the unknown can be a jarring experience if not approached with the appropriate level of care and attention. This is why middle school students need to be equipped with the fundamental knowledge necessary to excel in high school. Without proper preparation, the mere thought of moving from preschool to high school or college can spell disaster.

It is therefore imperative that students be given the tools and training they need to build a solid foundation upon which more complex concepts can be taught.

Similarly, shifting from a stable or even haphazard unhealthy eating system to a mindful nutritional system can prove challenging for the body, especially if the transitioning individual fails to prepare. So, it is crucial to make the switch to a healthier protocol as smooth as possible.

That way, the body will feel nourished rather than disgruntled due to the difficulties of adjusting to a new dietary plan.

All of the benefits that a healthy eating style brings to the individual are exhaustive. Having this consciousness and making the informed decision to aid your body through mindful eating requires some planning.

A businessman who takes on a project without forethought and reasonable groundwork could potentially set himself up for failure. So, to succeed in your journey and stick with it, you need knowledge of the main principles behind some lauded diets. So far, some of these principles have been discussed at great length. This is not a waste of time because accurate information lets you make dietary choices based on an informed understanding of what is best for you rather than jumping on every bandwagon.

To get started on this journey, you need to assess your current situation to be sure that it needs an upgrade. If you are faced with debilitating health conditions, this should be an inducement to get serious about a healthy transition. Your personal lifestyle inventory might also reveal unhealthy behaviors such as the overconsumption of processed foods, smoking, excessive alcohol intake, gluttony, and food binging.

These behaviors are capable of damaging the stability of the body and all of its regulators. When you discover an attunement to any of these or a slow slithering of these habits into your life, you have to gird yourself for change.

However, if your appraisal of present health conditions and habits indicates a measure of normality, you can still improve on what you already have by opting for any of the discussed dietary options.

What a healthy protocol means for you

A protocol is a recognized system of rules that guides an activity. So when we talk about a healthy dietary protocol, we are referring to a nutritive style that respects the accurate scientific recommendations for body nourishment. For instance, it is proven that inordinate amounts of processed food and sugar can be harmful to health, with research having linked these to cardiovascular diseases, diabetes, and other chronic diseases.

A healthy protocol will consider these standards while going a step further to make choices that are proven to manage and reverse the problems caused by ruinous habits.

Developing a healthy protocol involves a sweeping change in the way we function. It can sway from regulating sleeping patterns to adopting good nutritional plans, managing stress, and even establishing an exercise routine for wholesome living.

These factors are strongly linked to hormone function, so if you aim to regularize your hormone, you need to have a comprehensive plan that will address them.

To manage stress effectively, you have to review your daily activities to identify the ones that consume the larger percentage of your time and energy. You might have to reduce the length of time spent on such draining endeavors or even take some time off for quality rest.

For optimal health, experts recommend 7 to 9 hours of sleep for adults. Brain health is sustained this way, leading to a better quality of life.

Exercise is renewing physical activity that energizes the organs of the body and keeps them alert and ready to ward off health dangers. Because many adults have tight schedules that leave them with little or no time, exercising might be a challenge. If this is the case with you, you can still reach your exercise goal by dedicating 10 to 15 minutes early in the day for stretching and some light exercise.

Brisk walks and skipping can be done at home if you find that you are unable to go to the gymnasium. Furthermore, modern technology has seen a rise in exercise applications that are targeted at certain physical goals. You can download any of these on your mobile device and set reminders to avoid quitting. Overall, developing a regular schedule of exercise is necessary for sustained results.

Healthy transition guides

Making a smooth transition can start with setting a timeline for change. First, you can begin by introducing the new diet gradually into your eating plan. Let's say that you wish to adopt the ketogenic diet. A gradual change will mean that you do not cut off all carbohydrates in the beginning.

In the first week or two, you can choose to have a light ketogenic diet for breakfast, your normal carb diet for lunch, and another ketogenic diet for dinner eaten before 6 p.m. Next, you can introduce intermittent fasting to your routine before going all out on the ketogenic plan. Starting small and building momentum gives your body time to adapt to the new regimen and avoid shock.

Next, you need to build accountability and support systems that will help you on your journey. Support systems might be in the form of groups of people who have the same health goals and who are adopting the same dietary plan as yours.

These groups can be found in your immediate environment or online forums. Belonging to such communities will provide you with the daily motivation that you need to stay interested and focused on your given plan. Also, family and friends should be informed of your lifestyle change, and it will not be out of place to seek their support as you make certain modifications. When they see that you lack the drive or are beginning to lose interest, they could be the patrol guards that would jolt you back to the healthy course.

You might sometimes feel demotivated in your voyage toward better living because, as the saying goes, nothing good comes easy.

Setbacks could also arise when you cheat on your current plan. The goal, however, is to never remain down. When you notice that you seem to be going off track, try to get back on your journey without beating yourself up for the relapse. Reflecting on the future rewards will inspire you to persevere on this path and eventually develop a passion for it.

Another good way to excel is to anticipate common obstacles or roadblocks that might hinder your progress. Having a week- or month-long menu will enable you to plan adequately and avoid resorting to easily accessible meals that are not healthy. This may require that you have a sizable stock of raw food, for which you can keep regular logs to know when there is a need for a top-up.

You should also avoid the numerous social pressures that promote unhealthy foods. Televisions, social media, and shopping malls are saturated with promotions of processed foods, often disguised in nice packaging to attract buyers. A sure way to avoid these snares will be to master the act of controlling cravings. With the keto plan, this is easily achievable as the bulk of fatty foods is naturally designed to keep you full. Olive oil, nuts, and seeds are also constituents of Mediterranean meals with a reasonable fat content that can keep your cravings in check.

A healthy life is worth all the preliminary discomforts that come with adjusting what we were used to, to things that are edifying and designed to support robust health. In time, you will imbibe healthy habits and behaviors that will stay with you throughout your life. For every regular food out there, there is always a healthy alternative that can be given the same or better aesthetics.

A woman once felt that she would miss out on eating pancakes because of her new healthy dietary plan. I recommended that she prepares pancake but with healthy ingredients. Ingredients that could be used for this purpose include: oat flour, olive oil, plant-based milk, salt, and honey. Feel free to explore other recipes, and while you should adhere to your plan religiously, it would not be out of character to indulge your cravings for sweet things occasionally. However, you should apply care to this.

Stick to reliable measures of curtailing imbalances with diet

How do you feel when you attain milestones in life? I bet you are glad and eager to share your successes with loved ones. Making a change to a better diet plan can be counted as a milestone, and even more so is sticking to it. Nothing can be better than giving your life the gift of excellent nourishment. When your research leads you to settle on a plan or your nutritionist recommends one for you, adhering to it will be a huge relief to your organs.

In conclusion, every woman can optimize her hormone health and maintain an excellent body size by sticking to a stable diet plan. Mindful eating habits are powered by knowledge of evidence-based truths. It is important to note that the gap between intentional eaters and careless eaters is wide. While the latter predispose themselves to diseases, the former can hope to enjoy a healthy life relatively devoid of diseases.

Abnormal hormones set the body off on a chain of reactions that not only affect the vital organs but also impact social life and the physical body. Improve your chances of resolving common issues like fertility, premenopausal symptoms, acne, polycystic ovarian syndrome, obesity, fatigue, and mood swings by maintaining a good eating regimen.